S. R.

Healthy Dash Diet Recipes

First edition

This book was professionally typeset on Reedsy.
Find out more at reedsy.com

Contents

Contents

Chapter 1: Introduction

Welcome to the world of healthy eating! In this cookbook, you'll find a variety of tasty and nourishing recipes that are perfect for anyone looking to improve their diet and overall health. From grilled chicken Caesar salad and vegetarian chili to baked sweet potato fries and zucchini noodles with marinara sauce, there's something for everyone in this collection.

Whether you're trying to eat more vegetables, cut back on refined carbs, or just want to incorporate more healthy meals into your routine, these recipes are sure to hit the spot. They're easy to make and can be adapted to fit your specific dietary needs and preferences. So why wait? Start cooking up a storm and discover a new world of delicious and healthy meals that are sure to satisfy your cravings and nourish your body.

We hope you enjoy these recipes and that they inspire you to make healthy eating a part of your daily routine. Happy cooking!

Chapter 2: Grilled Chicken Caesar Salad

Ingredients:

4 chicken breasts

2 heads of romaine lettuce, chopped

2 cups plain Greek yogurt

2 tablespoons Dijon mustard

1 lemon, juiced

1 clove garlic, minced

Salt and pepper, to taste

Olive oil, for grilling

Instructions:

Preheat your grill to medium-high heat.

In a small bowl, mix together the Greek yogurt, Dijon mustard, lemon juice, minced garlic, salt, and pepper. Set aside.

Coat the chicken breasts with a small amount of olive oil and season with salt and pepper.

Place the chicken on the grill and cook for 6-8 minutes on each side, or until cooked through.

Remove the chicken from the grill and let it rest for a few minutes before slicing into thin strips.

In a large bowl, toss together the chopped romaine lettuce and grilled chicken strips.

Drizzle the Greek yogurt dressing over the top of the salad and toss to combine.

Serve the salad immediately, garnished with additional lemon wedges if desired.

Enjoy!

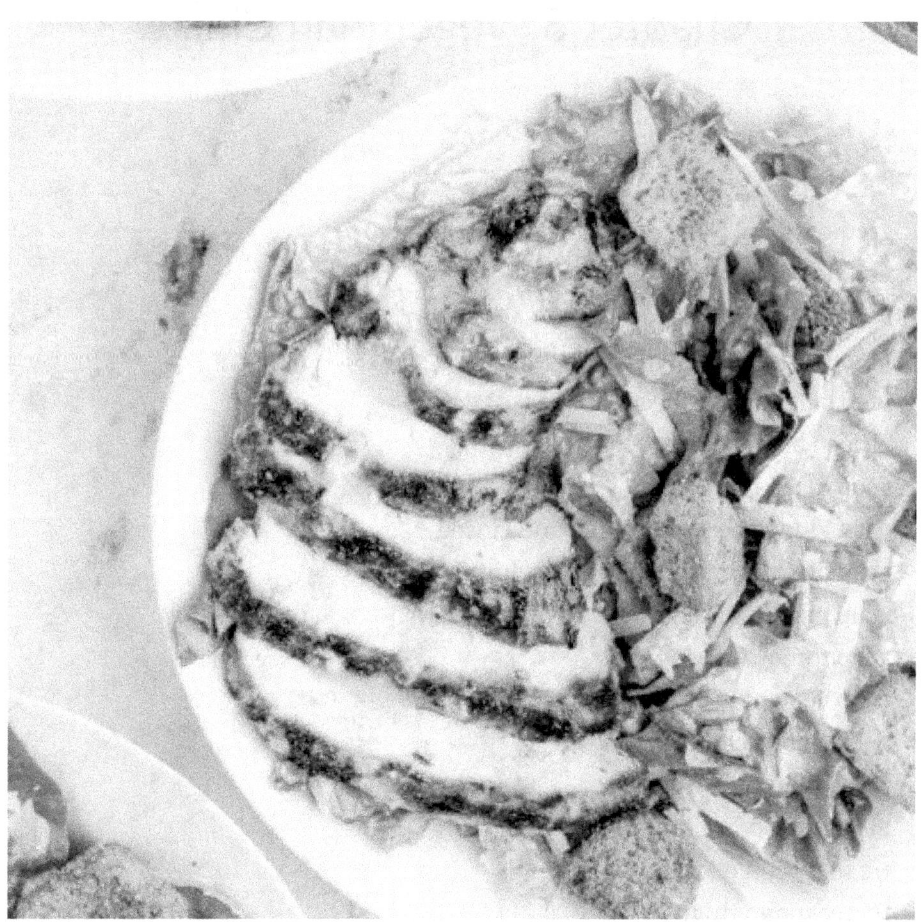

Chapter 3: Vegetarian Chili

Ingredients:

1 tablespoon olive oil

1 medium onion, diced

2 cloves garlic, minced

1 red bell pepper, diced

1 green bell pepper, diced

1 cup diced tomatoes

1 can kidney beans, drained and rinsed

1 can black beans, drained and rinsed

1 cup uncooked lentils

1 cup tomato sauce

1 cup vegetable broth

2 teaspoons chili powder

1 teaspoon cumin

1 teaspoon paprika

1/2 teaspoon oregano

1/2 teaspoon thyme

1/2 teaspoon salt

1/4 teaspoon black pepper

1 cup tofu, crumbled (optional)

Instructions:

In a large pot, heat the olive oil over medium heat. Add the onion and garlic and sauté for 5 minutes, until the onion is translucent.

Add the bell peppers, diced tomatoes, kidney beans, black beans, lentils, tomato sauce, vegetable broth, chili powder, cumin, paprika, oregano, thyme, salt, and black pepper to the pot. Stir to combine.

Bring the mixture to a boil, then reduce the heat to low and let it simmer for 30-40 minutes, or until the lentils are tender.

If using tofu, add it to the pot during the last 10 minutes of cooking.

Serve the chili hot, garnished with your choice of toppings such as shredded cheese, sour cream, and chopped scallions.

Enjoy!

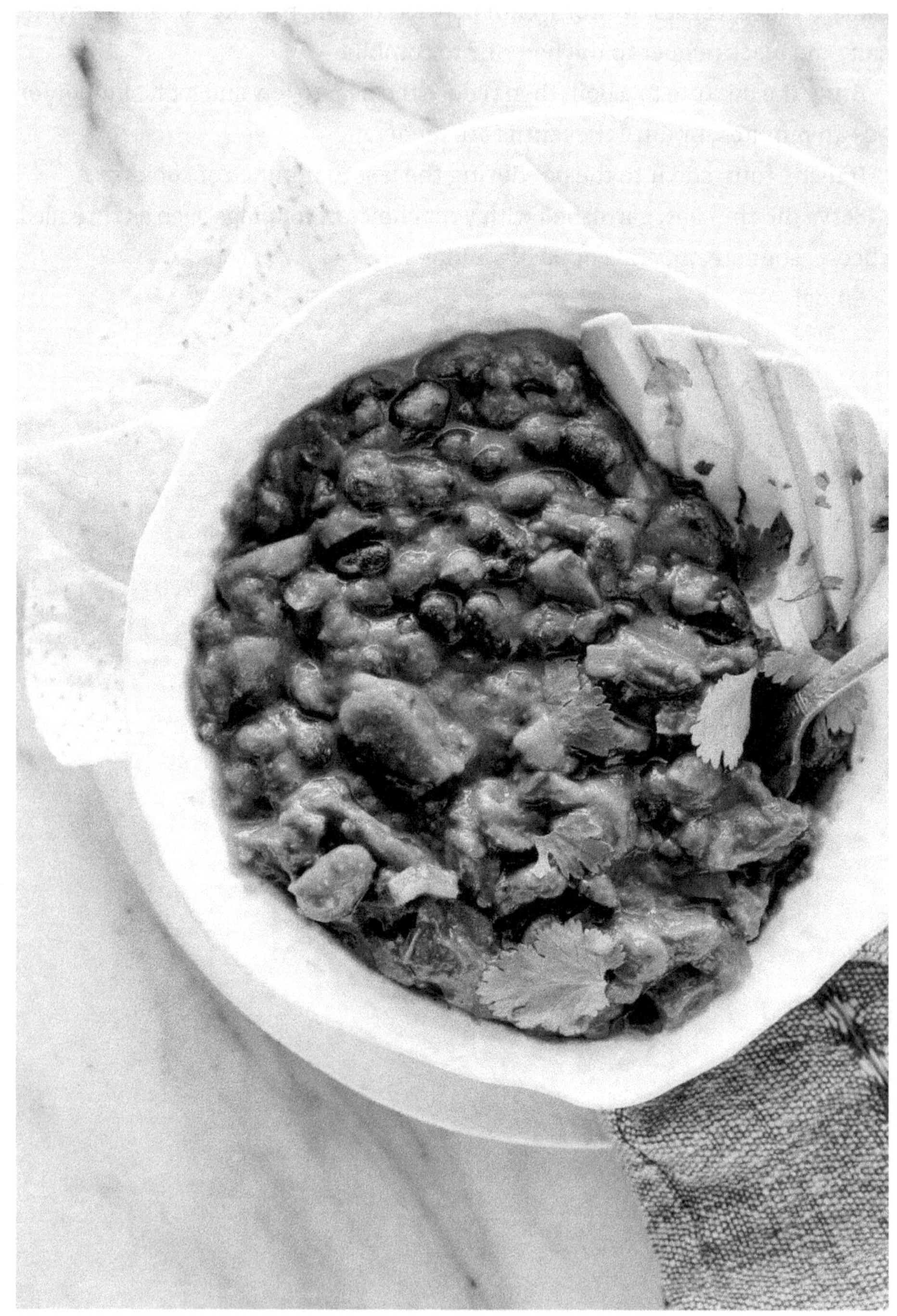

Chapter 4: Baked Sweet Potato Fries

Looking for a tasty and satisfying snack that won't derail your diet goals? Look no further than these baked sweet potato fries! They're a healthier alternative to traditional deep-fried fries, and they're bursting with flavor and nutrients. Plus, they're super easy to make - all you need is a few simple ingredients and an oven. Whether you're trying to eat more vegetables, cut back on refined carbs, or just want a tasty and satisfying snack, these baked sweet potato fries are sure to hit the spot. Try them out today and discover a new favorite snack that's both delicious and good for you!

Ingredients:

2 large sweet potatoes, peeled and cut into thin wedges

2 tablespoons olive oil

1 teaspoon salt

1 teaspoon paprika

1/2 teaspoon black pepper

1/2 teaspoon garlic powder

1/4 teaspoon onion powder

Instructions:

Preheat your oven to 425°F (220°C). Line a baking sheet with parchment paper.

In a large bowl, toss the sweet potato wedges with the olive oil, salt, paprika, black pepper, garlic powder, and onion powder.

Arrange the sweet potato wedges in a single layer on the prepared baking sheet.

Bake for 20-25 minutes, flipping the wedges halfway through, until they are tender and slightly crispy on the outside.

Serve the sweet potato fries hot, with a side of homemade guacamole or hummus for dipping.

Enjoy!

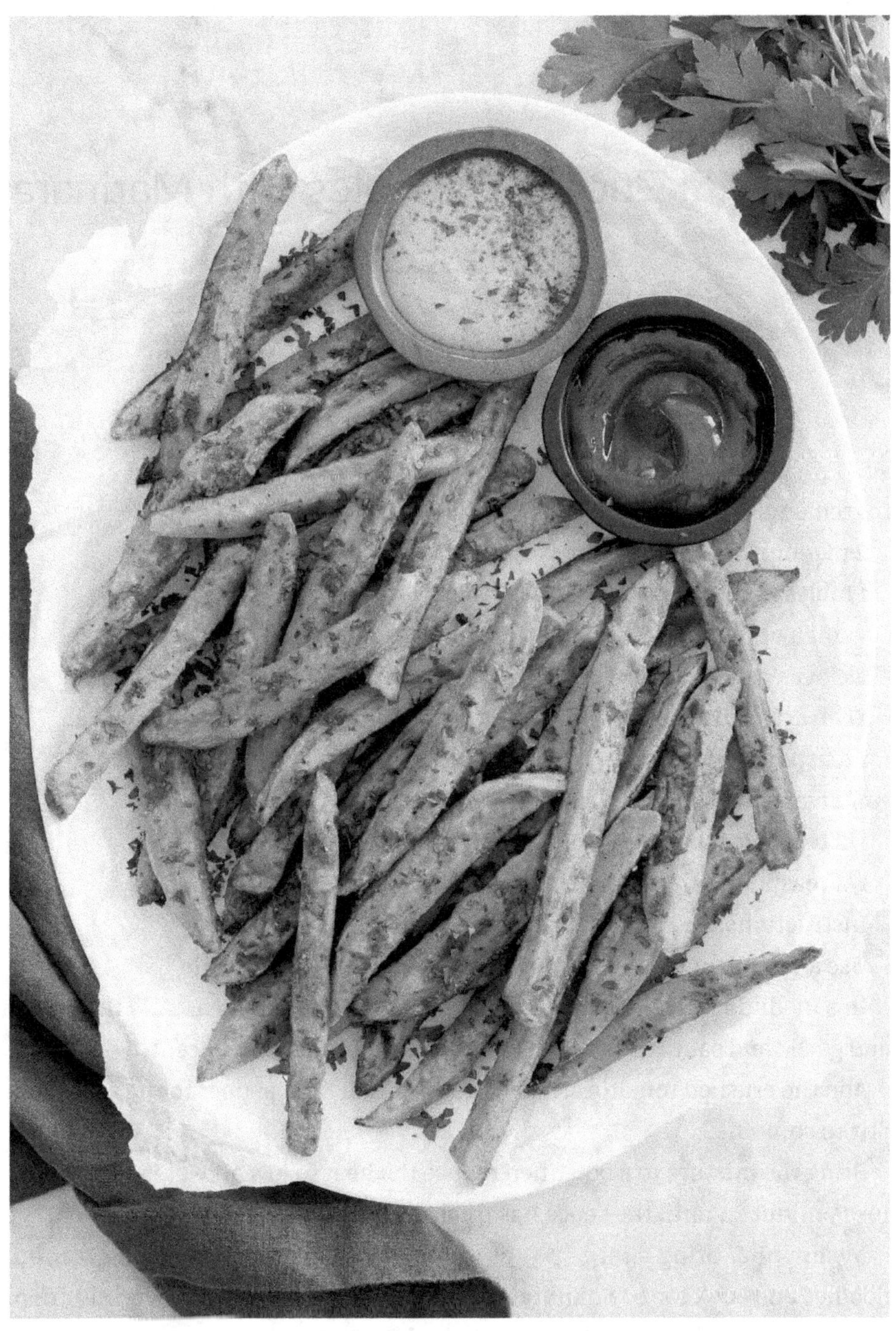

Chapter 5: Zucchini Noodles with Marinara Sauce

Ingredients:

2 medium zucchinis

1 tablespoon olive oil

1 small onion, diced

2 cloves garlic, minced

1 can crushed tomatoes

1 teaspoon dried basil

1/2 teaspoon dried oregano

1/2 teaspoon salt

1/4 teaspoon black pepper

Instructions:

Use a spiralizer to turn the zucchinis into noodles. Set aside.

In a medium saucepan, heat the olive oil over medium heat. Add the onion and garlic and sauté for 5 minutes, until the onion is translucent.

Add the crushed tomatoes, basil, oregano, salt, and pepper to the saucepan. Stir to combine.

Bring the mixture to a boil, then reduce the heat to low and let it simmer for 10-15 minutes, until the sauce has thickened slightly.

Meanwhile, bring a large pot of salted water to a boil. Add the zucchini noodles and cook for 2-3 minutes, until they are tender but still slightly crisp.

Drain the zucchini noodles and return them to the pot.

Pour the marinara sauce over the top of the noodles and toss to coat.

Serve the zucchini noodles hot, garnished with additional dried basil and Parmesan cheese if desired.

Enjoy!

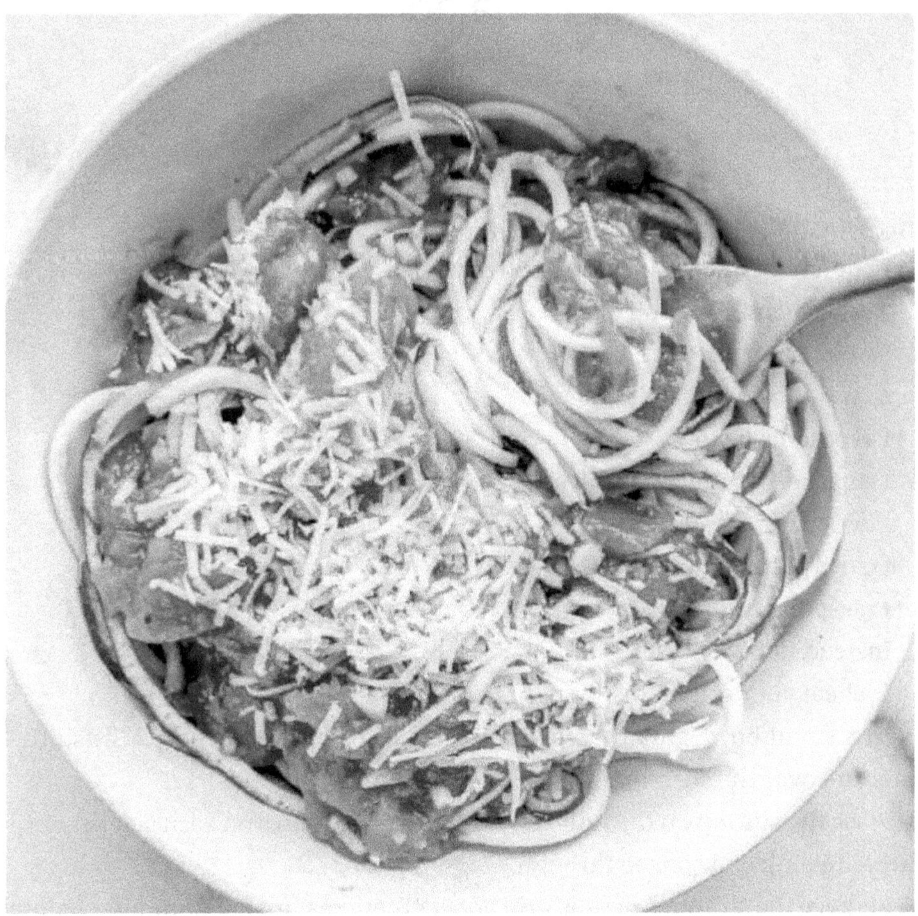

Chapter 6: Grilled Shrimp and Avocado Salad

Ingredients:

1 pound large shrimp, peeled and deveined

2 tablespoons olive oil

Salt and pepper, to taste

4 cups mixed greens

1 avocado, sliced

1 cup cherry tomatoes, halved

1 lemon, juiced

1 clove garlic, minced

1 teaspoon Dijon mustard

Instructions:

Preheat your grill to medium-high heat.

In a small bowl, mix together the olive oil, salt, and pepper. Brush the mixture over the shrimp.

Place the shrimp on the grill and cook for 2-3 minutes on each side, or until they are pink and cooked through.

Remove the shrimp from the grill and let them rest for a few minutes before slicing into bite-sized pieces.

In a small bowl, whisk together the lemon juice, minced garlic, Dijon mustard, and a pinch of salt. Slowly drizzle in the remaining olive oil, whisking constantly, until the dressing is emulsified.

In a large bowl, toss together the mixed greens, grilled shrimp, sliced avocado, and cherry tomatoes.

Drizzle the vinaigrette over the top of the salad and toss to combine.

Serve the salad immediately, garnished with additional lemon wedges if desired.

Enjoy!

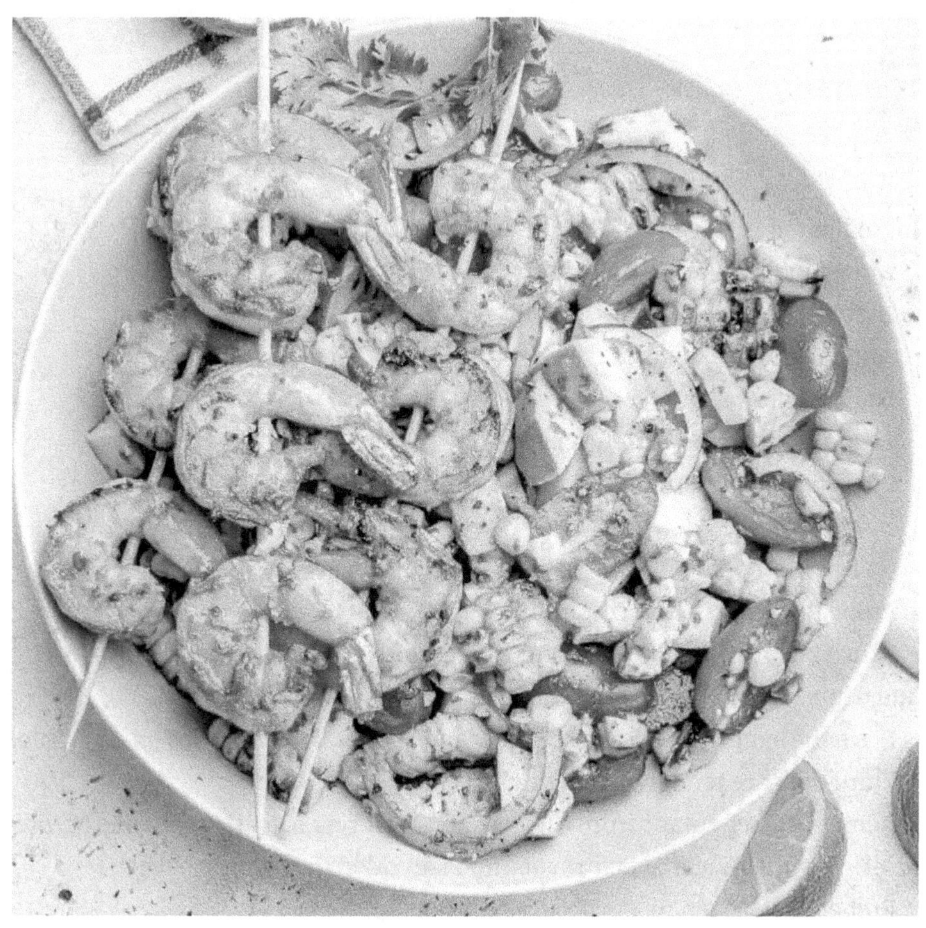

Chapter 7: Grilled or Baked Eggplant Parmesan

Ingredients:

2 medium eggplants, sliced into 1/4-inch rounds

2 tablespoons olive oil

Salt and pepper, to taste

1 cup marinara sauce

1 cup shredded mozzarella cheese

Fresh basil, for garnish

Instructions:

Grilled Method:

Preheat your grill to medium-high heat.

Brush both sides of the eggplant slices with olive oil and season with salt and pepper.

Place the eggplant slices on the grill and cook for 3-4 minutes on each side, or until they are tender and slightly charred.

Remove the eggplant from the grill and let it rest for a few minutes before layering it with the marinara sauce and shredded mozzarella cheese.

Preheat your oven to 350°F (180°C).

Place the eggplant slices in a single layer in a baking dish. Top each slice with a spoonful of marinara sauce and a sprinkle of mozzarella cheese.

Bake the eggplant parmesan for 10-15 minutes, or until the cheese is melted and bubbly.

Garnish the eggplant parmesan with fresh basil before serving.

Baked Method:

Preheat your oven to 400°F (200°C). Line a baking sheet with parchment paper.

Brush both sides of the eggplant slices with olive oil and season with salt and pepper.

Place the eggplant slices in a single layer on the prepared baking sheet.

Bake the eggplant for 15-20 minutes, or until it is tender and slightly browned.

Remove the eggplant from the oven and let it rest for a few minutes before layering it with the marinara sauce and shredded mozzarella cheese.

Preheat your oven to 350°F (180°C).

Place the eggplant slices in a single layer in a baking dish. Top each slice with a spoonful of marinara sauce and a sprinkle of mozzarella cheese.

Bake the eggplant parmesan for 10-15 minutes, or until the cheese is melted and bubbly.

Garnish the eggplant parmesan with fresh basil before serving.

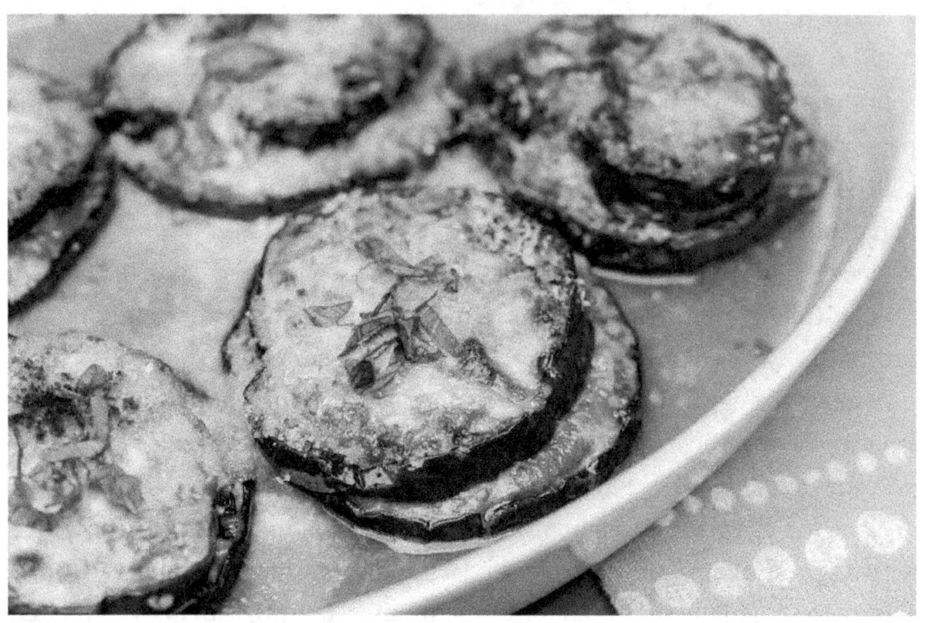

Chapter 8: Veggie and Hummus Wrap

Ingredients:

4 whole grain tortillas

1 cup hummus

1 cup mixed vegetables (such as bell peppers, cucumber, tomato, lettuce)

1/2 cup shredded cheese (optional)

Instructions:

Lay the tortillas out on a flat surface.

Spread a thin layer of hummus over each tortilla.

Arrange the mixed vegetables on top of the hummus.

If using cheese, sprinkle a small amount over the vegetables.

Roll up the tortillas tightly, making sure to tuck in the ends.

Slice the wraps into bite-sized pieces, if desired.

Serve the veggie and hummus wraps immediately, or wrap them in plastic wrap and refrigerate until ready to serve.

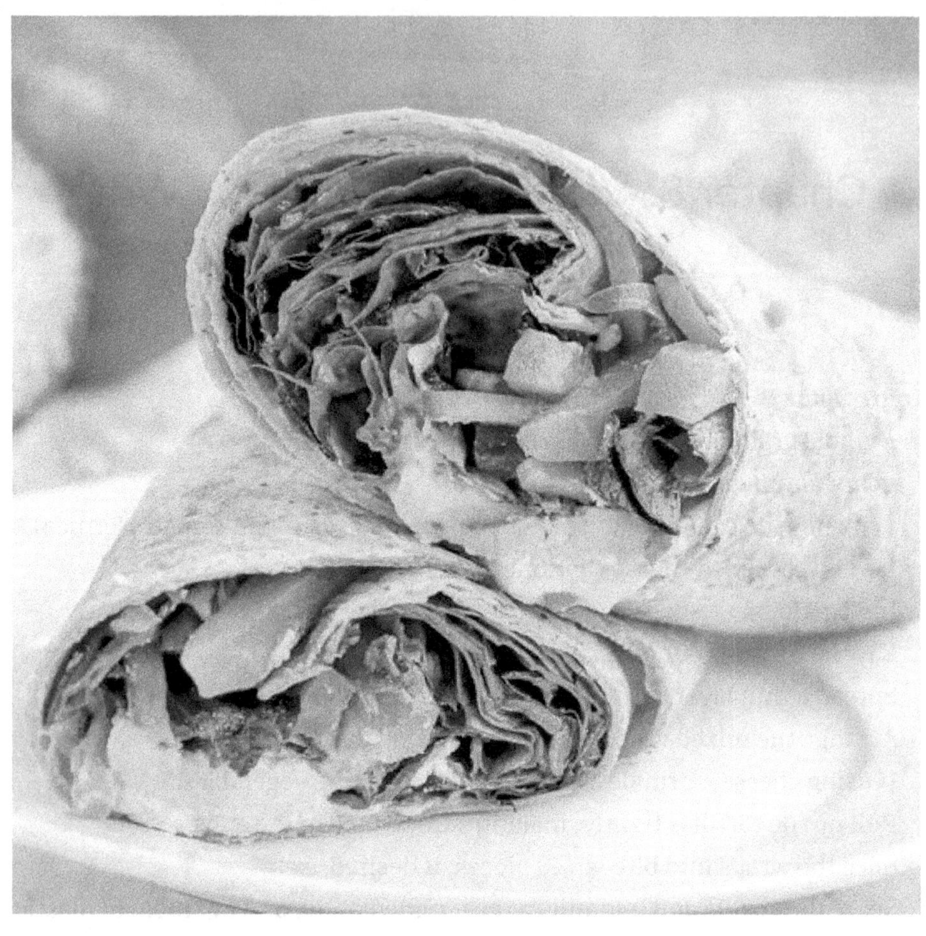

Chapter 9: Turkey and Spinach Meatballs

Get your protein fix and your daily serving of greens all in one bite with these flavorful and healthy turkey and spinach meatballs! Perfect for a quick and easy dinner or as a protein-packed snack on the go, these meatballs are sure to become a new family favorite

Ingredients:

1 pound ground turkey

1 cup finely chopped spinach

1/2 cup breadcrumbs

1 egg, beaten

1/2 teaspoon salt

1/4 teaspoon black pepper

1/4 teaspoon garlic powder

1/4 teaspoon onion powder

Instructions:

Preheat your oven to 400°F (200°C). Line a baking sheet with parchment paper.

In a large bowl, mix together the ground turkey, chopped spinach, breadcrumbs, egg, salt, pepper, garlic powder, and onion powder.

Use your hands to form the mixture into small meatballs, about 1-inch in diameter.

Place the meatballs on the prepared baking sheet and bake for 15-20 minutes, or until they are cooked through and browned on the outside.

Serve the turkey and spinach meatballs hot, with a side of whole grain pasta or spaghetti squash.

Enjoy!

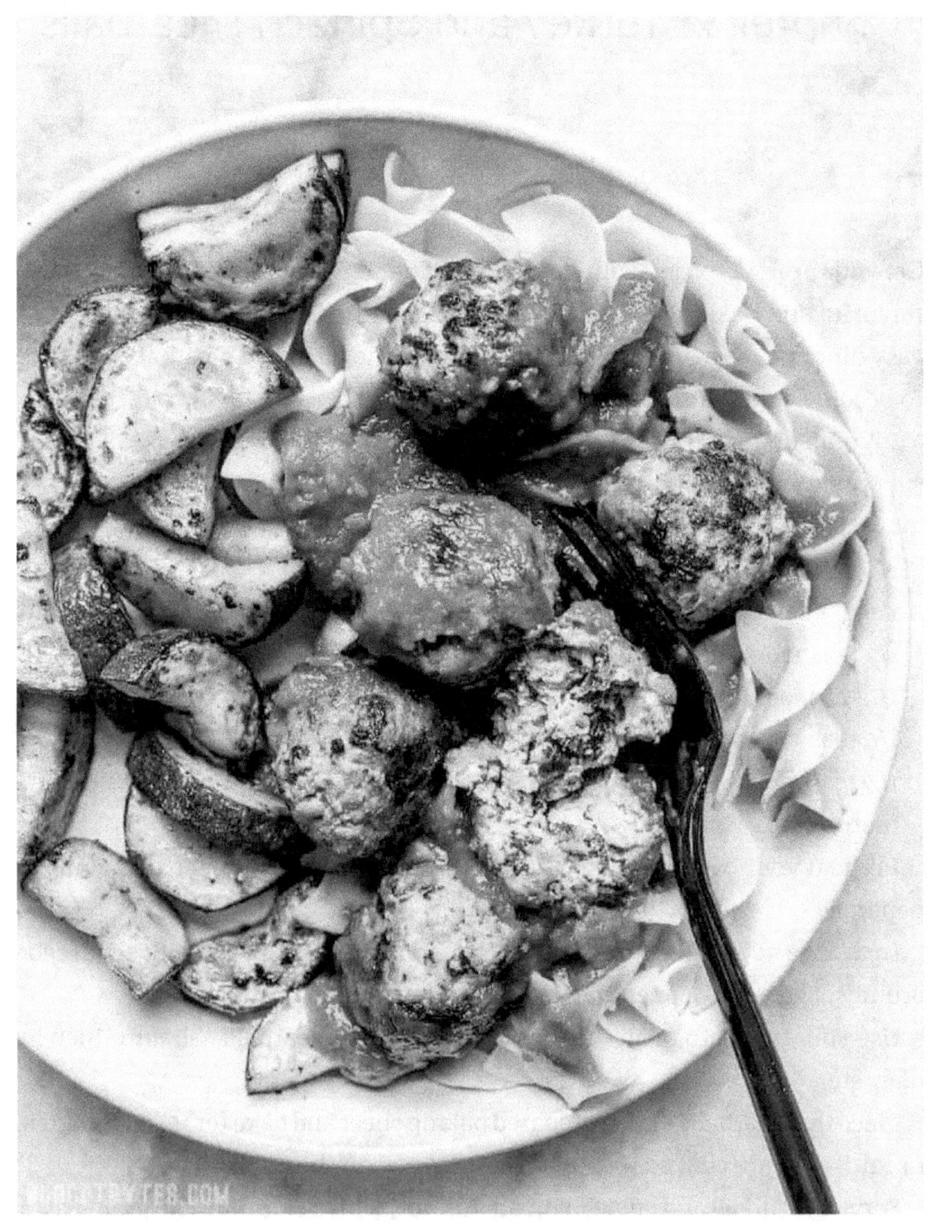

Chapter 10: Grilled Salmon and Vegetable Skewers

Ingredients:

1 pound salmon, cut into 1-inch chunks

1 red bell pepper, cut into 1-inch chunks

1 green bell pepper, cut into 1-inch chunks

1 medium onion, cut into 1-inch chunks

1 pint cherry tomatoes

2 tablespoons olive oil

Salt and pepper, to taste

Instructions:

Preheat your grill to medium-high heat.

Thread the salmon, bell peppers, onion, and cherry tomatoes onto skewers, alternating between the different ingredients.

Brush the skewers with olive oil and season with salt and pepper.

Place the skewers on the grill and cook for 8-10 minutes, turning occasionally, until the salmon is cooked through and the vegetables are tender.

Serve the grilled salmon and vegetable skewers hot, garnished with additional seasonings if desired.

Enjoy!

Chapter 11: Baked Falafel

Ingredients:

1 cup dried chickpeas, soaked in water overnight

1/2 cup chopped fresh parsley

1/2 cup chopped fresh cilantro

1 small onion, diced

3 cloves garlic, minced

1 teaspoon cumin

1 teaspoon coriander

1/2 teaspoon salt

1/4 teaspoon black pepper

2 tablespoons all-purpose flour

Olive oil, for baking

Instructions:

Preheat your oven to 400°F (200°C). Line a baking sheet with parchment paper.

Drain and rinse the soaked chickpeas, then place them in a food processor along with the parsley, cilantro, onion, garlic, cumin, coriander, salt, and pepper. Pulse the mixture until it is well combined and slightly chunky.

Transfer the mixture to a large bowl and mix in the flour until well combined.

Use your hands to shape the mixture into small balls, about 1-inch in diameter. Place the balls on the prepared baking sheet.

Lightly brush the tops of the falafel balls with olive oil.

Bake the falafel for 15-20 minutes, or until they are browned and crispy on the outside.

Serve the baked falafel hot, with a side of tzatziki sauce or your favorite dipping sauce.

Enjoy!

Chapter 12: Mushroom and Asparagus Stir-Fry

Ingredients:

1 pound sliced mushrooms

1 pound asparagus, cut into 1-inch pieces

2 tablespoons vegetable oil

3 cloves garlic, minced

1/2 cup stir-fry sauce

4 cups cooked brown rice or quinoa, for serving

Instructions:

Heat a large wok or frying pan over medium-high heat. Add the vegetable oil and swirl to coat the pan.

Add the sliced mushrooms and asparagus to the pan and sauté for 5-7 minutes, or until the vegetables are tender.

Add the minced garlic and stir-fry sauce to the pan and stir to coat the vegetables.

Cook for an additional 2-3 minutes, or until the sauce is heated through.

Serve the mushroom and asparagus stir-fry over a bed of cooked brown rice or quinoa.

Enjoy!

Chapter 13: Avocado and Black Bean Quesadillas

Ingredients:

2 whole grain tortillas

1 avocado, mashed

1 cup black beans, rinsed and drained

1/2 cup shredded cheese

Olive oil, for grilling

Instructions:

Lay the tortillas out on a flat surface.

Spread the mashed avocado over one half of each tortilla, leaving a small border around the edges.

Top the avocado with the black beans and shredded cheese.

Fold the tortillas in half, pressing gently to seal.

Heat a large frying pan over medium heat. Add a small amount of olive oil to the pan and swirl to coat.

Place the quesadillas in the pan and cook for 2-3 minutes on each side, or until the cheese is melted and the tortillas are crispy.

Cut the quesadillas into wedges and serve hot, with a side of salsa or sour cream for dipping.

Enjoy!

Chapter 14: Grilled Vegetable and Goat Cheese Salad

Looking for a delicious and healthy way to incorporate more vegetables into your diet? Look no further than this grilled vegetable and goat cheese salad! Packed with a variety of grilled vegetables and creamy goat cheese, this salad is bursting with flavor and nutrients. Plus, it's super easy to make and can be served as a main course or as a side dish. Whether you're trying to eat more vegetables, cut back on meat, or just want a tasty and satisfying meal, this grilled vegetable and goat cheese salad is sure to hit the spot. So fire up the grill and give this recipe a try today!

Ingredients:

1 small eggplant, cut into 1/2-inch slices
1 red bell pepper, cut into 1/2-inch slices
1 green bell pepper, cut into 1/2-inch slices
1 medium zucchini, cut into 1/2-inch slices
2 tablespoons olive oil
Salt and pepper, to taste
4 cups mixed greens
1/2 cup crumbled goat cheese
1 lemon, juiced
1 clove garlic, minced
1 teaspoon Dijon mustard

Instructions:

Preheat your grill to medium-high heat.

Brush both sides of the eggplant, bell pepper, and zucchini slices with olive oil and season with salt and pepper.

Place the vegetables on the grill and cook for 3-4 minutes on each side, or until they are tender and slightly charred.

Remove the vegetables from the grill and let them rest for a few minutes before slicing them into bite-sized pieces.

In a small bowl, whisk together the lemon juice, minced garlic, Dijon mustard, and a pinch of salt. Slowly drizzle in the remaining olive oil, whisking constantly, until the dressing is emulsified.

In a large bowl, toss together the mixed greens, grilled

Chapter 15: Spaghetti Squash with Marinara Sauce

Ingredients:

1 medium spaghetti squash

2 tablespoons olive oil

Salt and pepper, to taste

1 small onion, diced

2 cloves garlic, minced

1 can crushed tomatoes

1 teaspoon dried basil

1/2 teaspoon dried oregano

1/2 teaspoon salt

1/4 teaspoon black pepper

1 cup crumbled tofu or diced tempeh (optional)

Instructions:

Preheat your oven to 400°F (200°C). Line a baking sheet with parchment paper.

Cut the spaghetti squash in half lengthwise and scoop out the seeds.

Brush the cut sides of the squash with olive oil and season with salt and pepper.

Place the squash cut-side down on the prepared baking sheet.

Bake the squash for 30-40 minutes, or until it is tender and the flesh can be easily shredded with a fork.

Remove the squash from the oven and let it cool for a few minutes.

Use a fork to shred the squash into "noodles" and set aside.

In a medium saucepan, heat the remaining olive oil over medium heat. Add the onion and garlic and sauté for 5 minutes, until the onion is translucent.

Add the crushed tomatoes, basil, oregano, salt, and pepper to the saucepan. Stir to combine.

If using tofu or tempeh, add it to the saucepan and stir to combine.

Bring the mixture to a boil, then reduce the heat to low and let it simmer for 10-15 minutes, until the sauce has thickened slightly.

Meanwhile, bring a large pot of salted water to a boil. Add the spaghetti squash noodles and cook for 2-3 minutes, until they are tender but still slightly crisp.

Drain the spaghetti squash noodles and return them to the pot.

Pour the marinara sauce over the top of the noodles and toss to coat.

Serve the spaghetti squash hot, garnished with additional dried basil and Parmesan cheese if desired.

Enjoy!

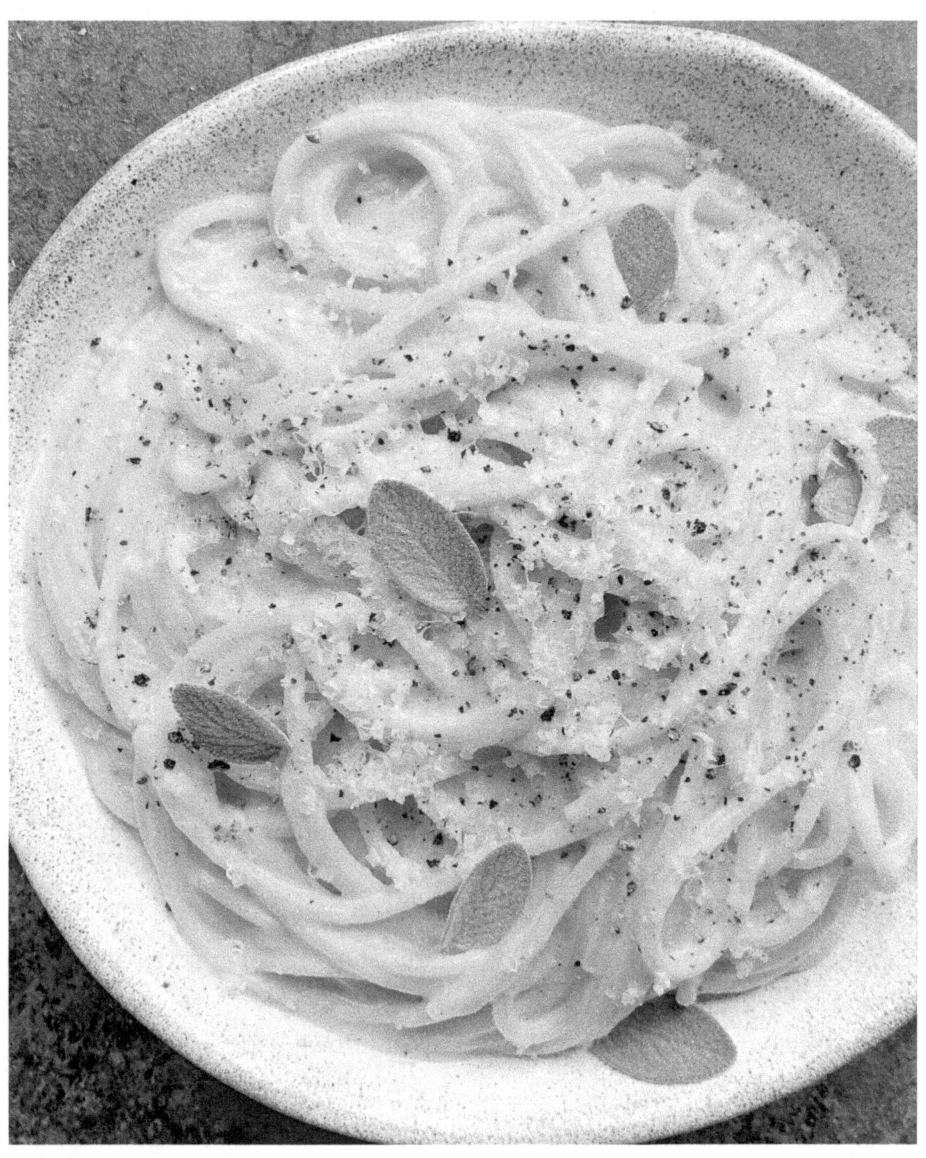

Chapter 16:

Cauliflower Crust Pizza

Ingredients:

1 small head of cauliflower, grated

1 egg

1/2 cup shredded cheese (such as mozzarella or cheddar)

1/4 cup all-purpose flour

1/4 teaspoon salt

1/4 teaspoon black pepper

1 cup tomato sauce

1 cup chopped vegetables (such as bell peppers, onions, mushrooms)

Additional shredded cheese, for topping

Instructions:

Preheat your oven to 400°F (200°C). Line a baking sheet with parchment paper.

In a large bowl, mix together the grated cauliflower, egg, 1/2 cup of cheese, flour, salt, and pepper.

Press the mixture into a thin, even layer on the prepared baking sheet.

Bake the cauliflower crust for 20-25 minutes, or until it is firm and golden brown.

Remove the crust from the oven and let it cool for a few minutes.

Spread the tomato sauce over the crust, leaving a small border around the edges.

Top the sauce with the chopped vegetables and a sprinkle of additional cheese.

Return the pizza to the oven and bake for an additional 10-15 minutes, or until the cheese is melted and bubbly.

Serve the cauliflower crust pizza hot, garnished with fresh herbs if desired.

Enjoy!

Chapter 17: Baked Chicken and Vegetable Fajitas

Ingredients:

1 pound chicken breasts

1/4 cup lime juice

2 cloves garlic, minced

1 teaspoon cumin

1 teaspoon chili powder

1/2 teaspoon paprika

1/4 teaspoon salt

1/4 teaspoon black pepper

1 red bell pepper, sliced

1 green bell pepper, sliced

1 medium onion, sliced

2 tablespoons olive oil

8 whole grain tortillas

Instructions:

Preheat your oven to 400°F (200°C). Line a baking sheet with parchment paper.

In a small bowl, mix together the lime juice, garlic, cumin, chili powder, paprika, salt, and pepper.

Place the chicken breasts in a shallow dish and pour the marinade over the top. Let the chicken marinate for at least 20 minutes, or up to 4 hours.

Place the chicken on the prepared baking sheet and bake for 20-25 minutes, or until it is cooked through and the internal temperature reaches 165°F (75°C).

Remove the chicken from the oven and let it rest for a few minutes before slicing it into thin strips.

In a large frying pan, heat the olive oil over medium-high heat. Add the bell peppers and onion and sauté for 5-7 minutes, or until they are tender.

Add the sliced chicken to the pan and stir to combine.

Warm the tortillas in the microwave or on a griddle.

To assemble the fajitas, place a small amount of the chicken and vegetable mixture in the center of each tortilla. Top with desired toppings such as salsa, sour cream, and shredded cheese.

Fold the tortillas in half and serve the fajitas hot.

Enjoy!

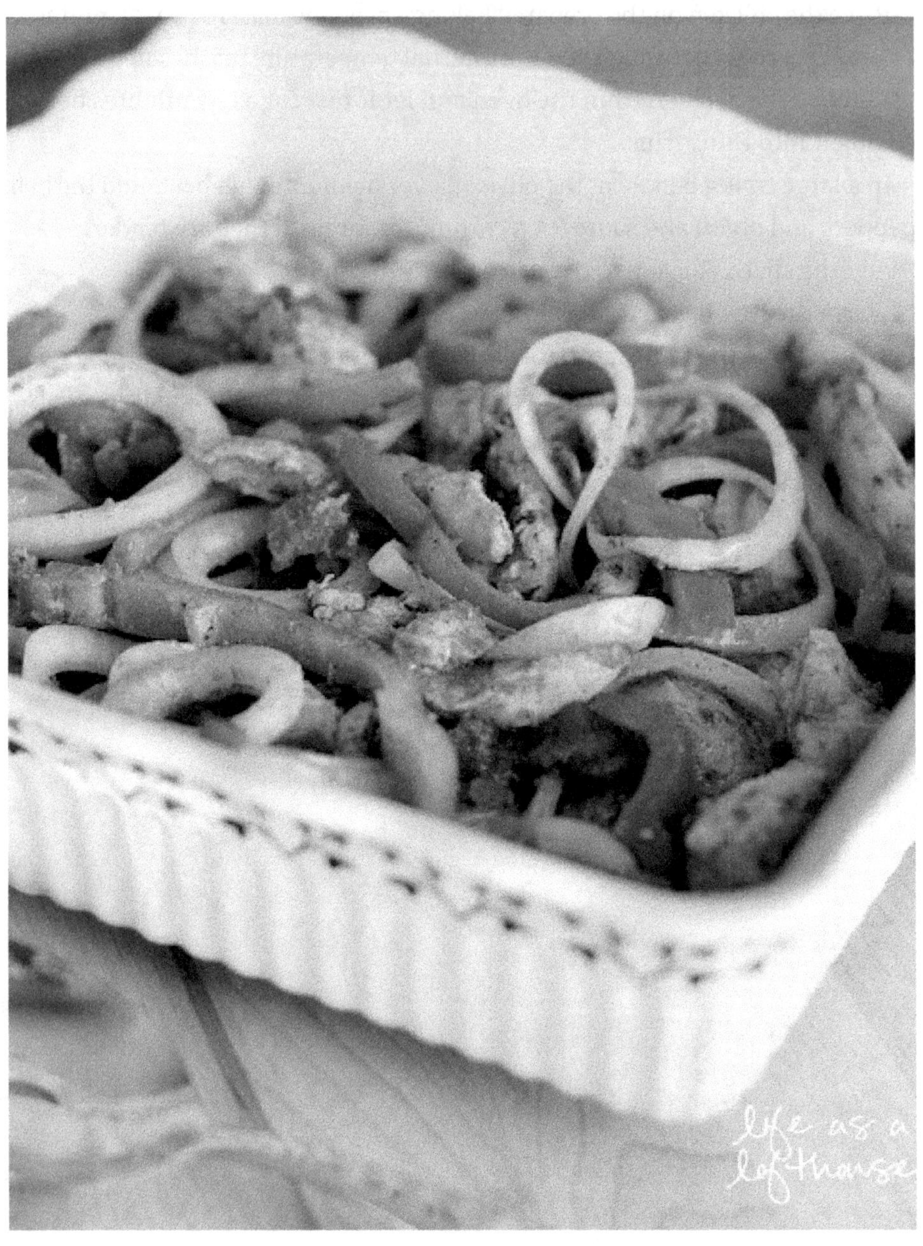
life as a
lofthouse

Chapter 18: Grilled Salmon and Quinoa Bowl

Ingredients:

1 pound salmon fillets

2 cups cooked quinoa

2 cups mixed roasted vegetables (such as bell peppers, onions, and cherry tomatoes)

1 lemon, juiced

2 tablespoons olive oil

1 clove garlic, minced

Salt and pepper, to taste

Instructions:

Preheat your grill to medium-high heat.

Season the salmon fillets with salt and pepper.

Place the salmon on the grill and cook for 8-10 minutes, turning once, until it is cooked through and flakes easily with a fork.

Remove the salmon from the grill and let it rest for a few minutes before slicing it into bite-sized pieces.

In a small bowl, whisk together the lemon juice, olive oil, minced garlic, and a pinch of salt.

In a large bowl, toss together the cooked quinoa, roasted vegetables, and sliced salmon.

Drizzle the citrus vinaigrette over the top of the quinoa bowl and toss to coat.

Serve the grilled salmon and quinoa bowl hot, garnished with additional chopped herbs if desired.

Enjoy!

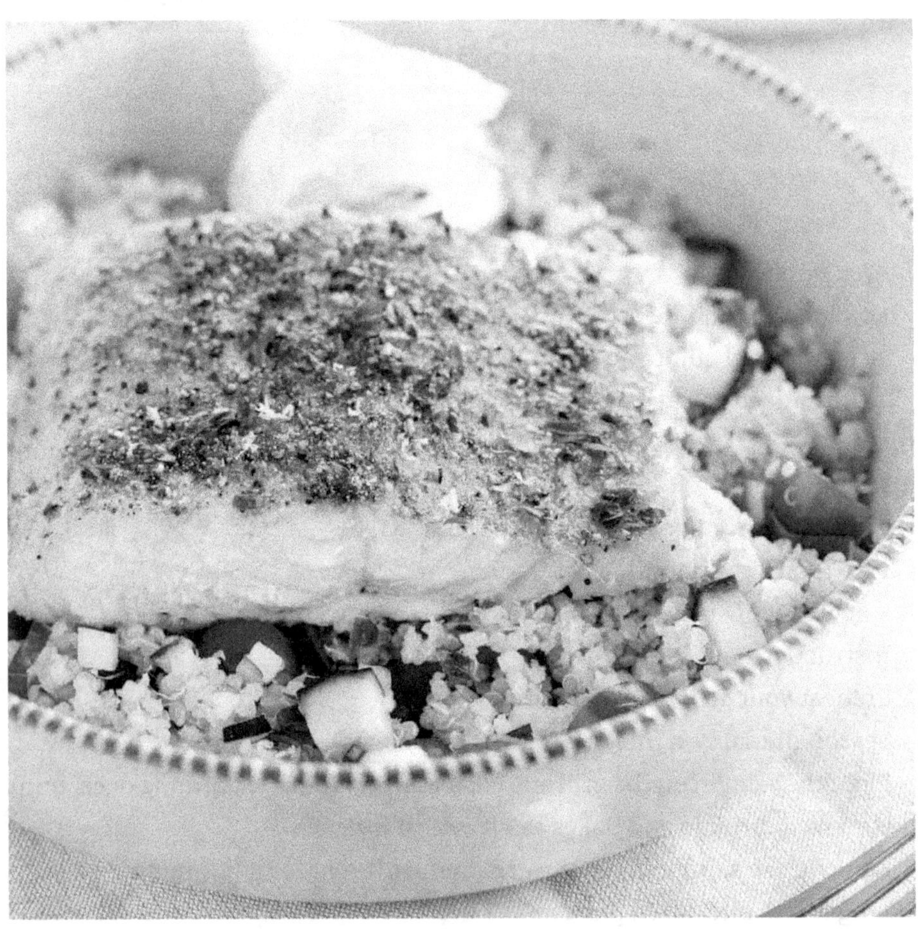

Chapter 19: Stuffed Peppers

Ingredients:

4 large bell peppers

1 cup cooked quinoa

1 cup diced vegetables (such as bell peppers, onions, and tomatoes)

1/2 cup shredded cheese (such as mozzarella or cheddar)

1 tablespoon olive oil

1 clove garlic, minced

1/2 teaspoon salt

1/4 teaspoon black pepper

Instructions:

Preheat your oven to 400°F (200°C). Line a baking sheet with parchment paper.

Cut the bell peppers in half lengthwise and remove the seeds and stem.

In a large bowl, mix together the cooked quinoa, diced vegetables, shredded cheese, olive oil, minced garlic, salt, and pepper.

Spoon the mixture into the cavity of the bell pepper halves, dividing it evenly between the peppers.

Place the stuffed peppers on the prepared baking sheet.

Bake the peppers for 20-25 minutes, or until they are tender and the filling is hot.

Serve the stuffed peppers hot, garnished with additional cheese and fresh herbs if desired.

Enjoy!

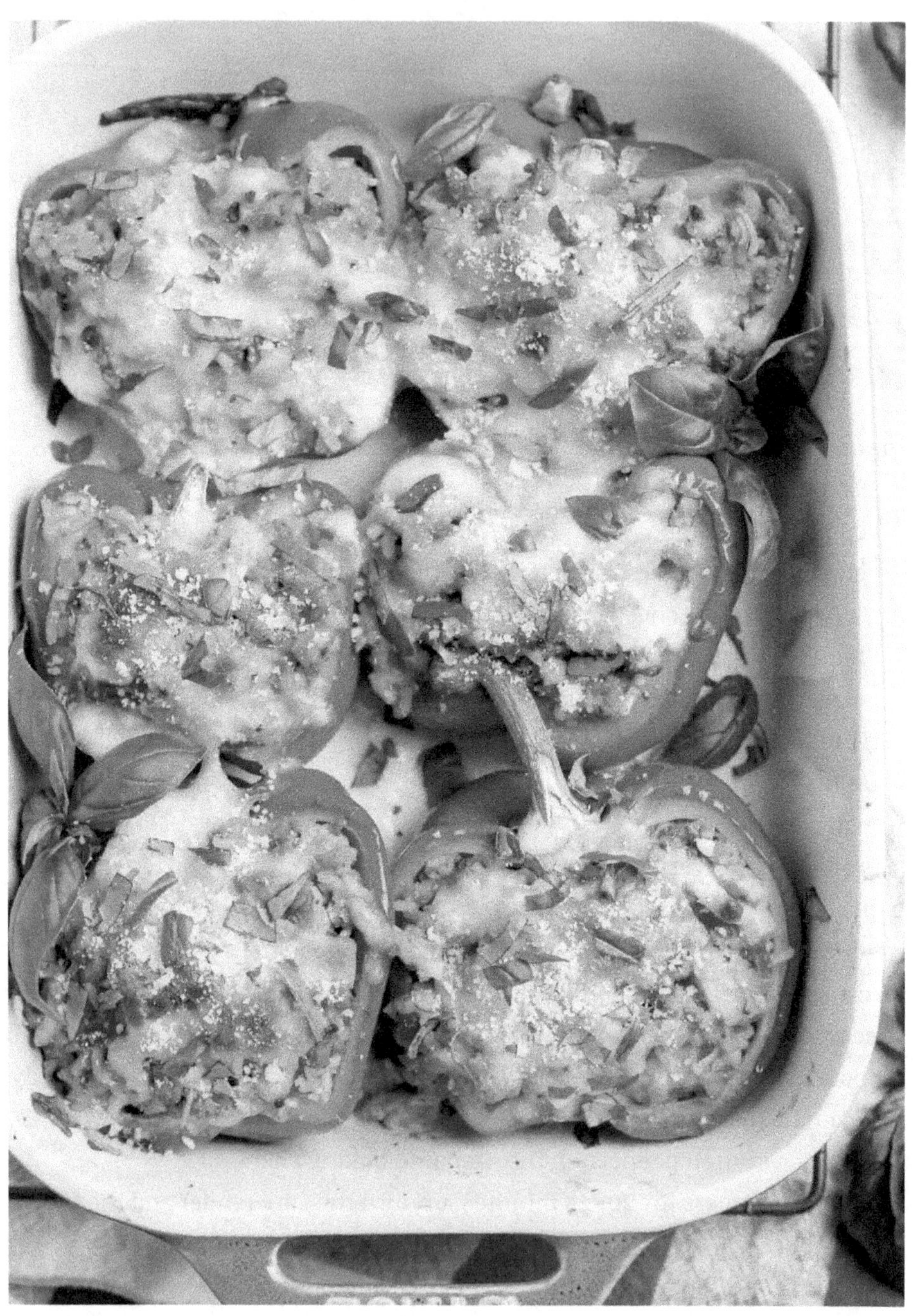

Chapter 20: Grilled Chicken and Avocado Salad

Ingredients:

1 pound chicken breasts

4 cups mixed greens

1 avocado, sliced

1 cup cherry tomatoes, halved

1 lemon, juiced

2 tablespoons olive oil

1 clove garlic, minced

Salt and pepper, to taste

Instructions:

Preheat your grill to medium-high heat.

Season the chicken breasts with salt and pepper.

Place the chicken on the grill and cook for 8-10 minutes, turning once, until it is cooked through and the internal temperature reaches 165°F (75°C).

Remove the chicken from the grill and let it rest for a few minutes before slicing it into thin strips.

In a small bowl, whisk together the lemon juice, olive oil, minced garlic, and a pinch of salt.

In a large bowl, toss together the mixed greens, sliced avocado, cherry tomatoes, and sliced chicken.

Drizzle the vinaigrette over the top of the salad and toss to coat.

Serve the grilled chicken and avocado salad hot, garnished with additional chopped herbs if desired.

Enjoy!

Chapter 21: Baked Sweet Potato and Black Bean Burritos with Grilled Chicken

Ingredients:

1 pound chicken breasts

2 large sweet potatoes, peeled and diced

1 can black beans, rinsed and drained

1 cup diced vegetables (such as bell peppers, onions, and tomatoes)

1 cup shredded cheese (such as mozzarella or cheddar)

8 whole grain tortillas

Olive oil, for grilling

Salt and pepper, to taste

Instructions:

Preheat your grill to medium-high heat.

Season the chicken breasts with salt and pepper.

Place the chicken on the grill and cook for 8-10 minutes, turning once, until it is cooked through and the internal temperature reaches 165°F (75°C).

Remove the chicken from the grill and let it rest for a few minutes before slicing it into thin strips.

In the meantime, bring a large pot of salted water to a boil. Add the sweet potatoes and cook for 8-10 minutes, or until they are tender.

Drain the sweet potatoes and mash them with a potato masher or fork.

In a large bowl, mix together the mashed sweet potatoes, black beans, diced vegetables, and shredded cheese.

Preheat your oven to 350°F (180°C). Line a baking sheet with parchment paper.

Lay the tortillas out on a flat surface. Divide the sweet potato and black bean mixture evenly between the tortillas, placing it in the center of each tortilla. Top the mixture with sliced grilled chicken.

Fold the sides of the tortillas over the filling and roll them up tightly. Place the burritos seam-side down on the prepared baking sheet.

Bake the burritos for 10-15 minutes, or until they are heated through and the cheese is melted.

Serve the baked sweet potato and black bean burritos hot, garnished with additional diced vegetables and cheese

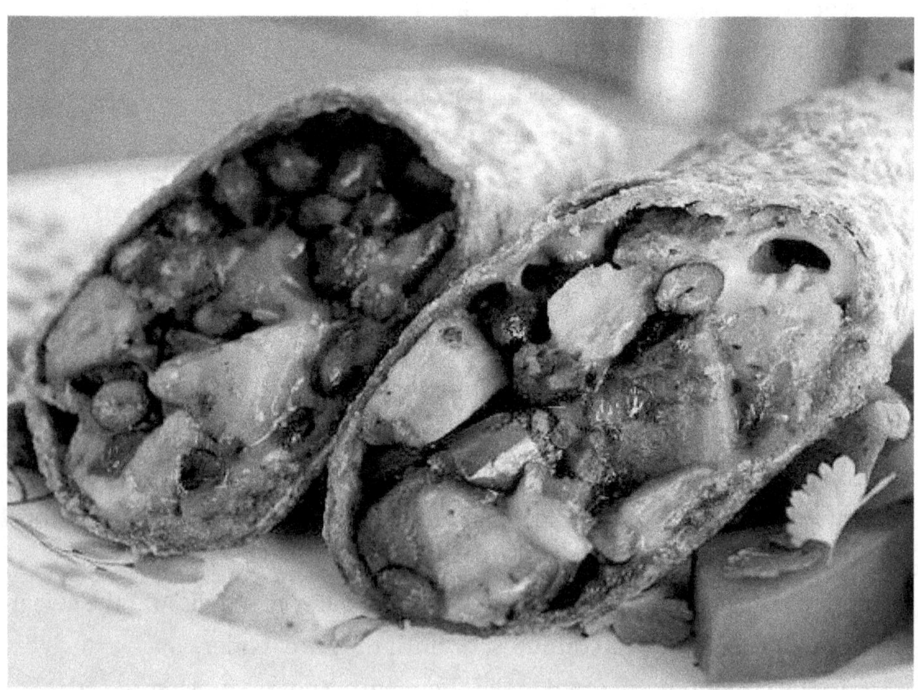

Chapter 21: Grilled Vegetable and Hummus Wrap

Ingredients:

1 medium eggplant, sliced into 1/4-inch rounds

1 red bell pepper, sliced into 1/4-inch strips

1 green bell pepper, sliced into 1/4-inch strips

1 zucchini, sliced into 1/4-inch rounds

Olive oil, for grilling

Salt and pepper, to taste

4 whole grain tortillas

1 cup hummus

4 lettuce leaves

Instructions:

Preheat your grill to medium-high heat.

Brush the eggplant, bell peppers, and zucchini slices with a small amount of olive oil and season with salt and pepper.

Place the vegetables on the grill and cook for 5-7 minutes on each side, or until they are tender and grill marks appear.

Remove the vegetables from the grill and let them cool for a few minutes.

Lay the tortillas out on a flat surface. Spread a spoonful of hummus onto the center of each tortilla.

Top the hummus with a lettuce leaf and a small amount of grilled vegetables.

Fold the sides of the tortillas over the filling and roll them up tightly.

Serve the grilled vegetable and hummus wraps hot, garnished with additional diced vegetables and hummus if desired.

Enjoy!

Chapter 22: Grilled Eggplant and Tomato Salad

Ingredients:

1 medium eggplant, sliced into 1/4-inch rounds

Olive oil, for grilling

Salt and pepper, to taste

4 cups mixed greens

2 medium tomatoes, sliced

2 tablespoons lemon juice

2 tablespoons olive oil

1 clove garlic, minced

Salt and pepper, to taste

Instructions:

Preheat your grill to medium-high heat.

Brush the eggplant slices with a small amount of olive oil and season with salt and pepper.

Place the eggplant on the grill and cook for 5-7 minutes on each side, or until it is tender and grill marks appear.

Remove the eggplant from the grill and let it cool for a few minutes.

In a small bowl, whisk together the lemon juice, 2 tablespoons of olive oil, minced garlic, and a pinch of salt and pepper.

In a large bowl, toss together the mixed greens, sliced tomatoes, and grilled eggplant.

Drizzle the vinaigrette over the top of the salad and toss to coat.

Serve the grilled eggplant and tomato salad hot, garnished with additional chopped herbs if desired.

Enjoy!

Chapter 23: Baked Falafel Bowls

Ingredients:

1 cup dry chickpeas, soaked in water overnight

1/4 cup fresh parsley, chopped

1/4 cup fresh cilantro, chopped

1 clove garlic, minced

1/2 medium onion, finely chopped

1 teaspoon cumin

1 teaspoon coriander

1/2 teaspoon salt

1/4 teaspoon black pepper

2 tablespoons all-purpose flour

Olive oil, for baking

2 cups cooked quinoa

2 cups mixed roasted vegetables (such as bell peppers, onions, and cherry tomatoes)

1 cup Greek yogurt

1 lemon, juiced

1 small cucumber, grated

Salt and pepper, to taste

Instructions:

Preheat your oven to 400°F (200°C). Line a baking sheet with parchment paper.

Drain and rinse the soaked chickpeas. Place them in a food processor with the parsley, cilantro, garlic, onion, cumin, coriander, salt, and pepper. Pulse until the mixture is well combined and forms a rough paste.

Transfer the chickpea mixture to a large bowl and stir in the flour.

Using wet hands, shape the mixture into small balls and place them on the prepared baking sheet.

Brush the falafel balls with a small amount of olive oil.

Bake the falafel for 15-20 minutes, or until they are golden brown and crisp on the outside.

In a small bowl, mix together the Greek yogurt, lemon juice, grated cucumber, and a pinch of salt and pepper.

To assemble the falafel bowls, place a small amount of cooked quinoa in the bottom of each bowl. Top the quinoa with roasted vegetables and baked falafel.

Serve the falafel bowls with a side of tzatziki sauce for dipping.

Enjoy!

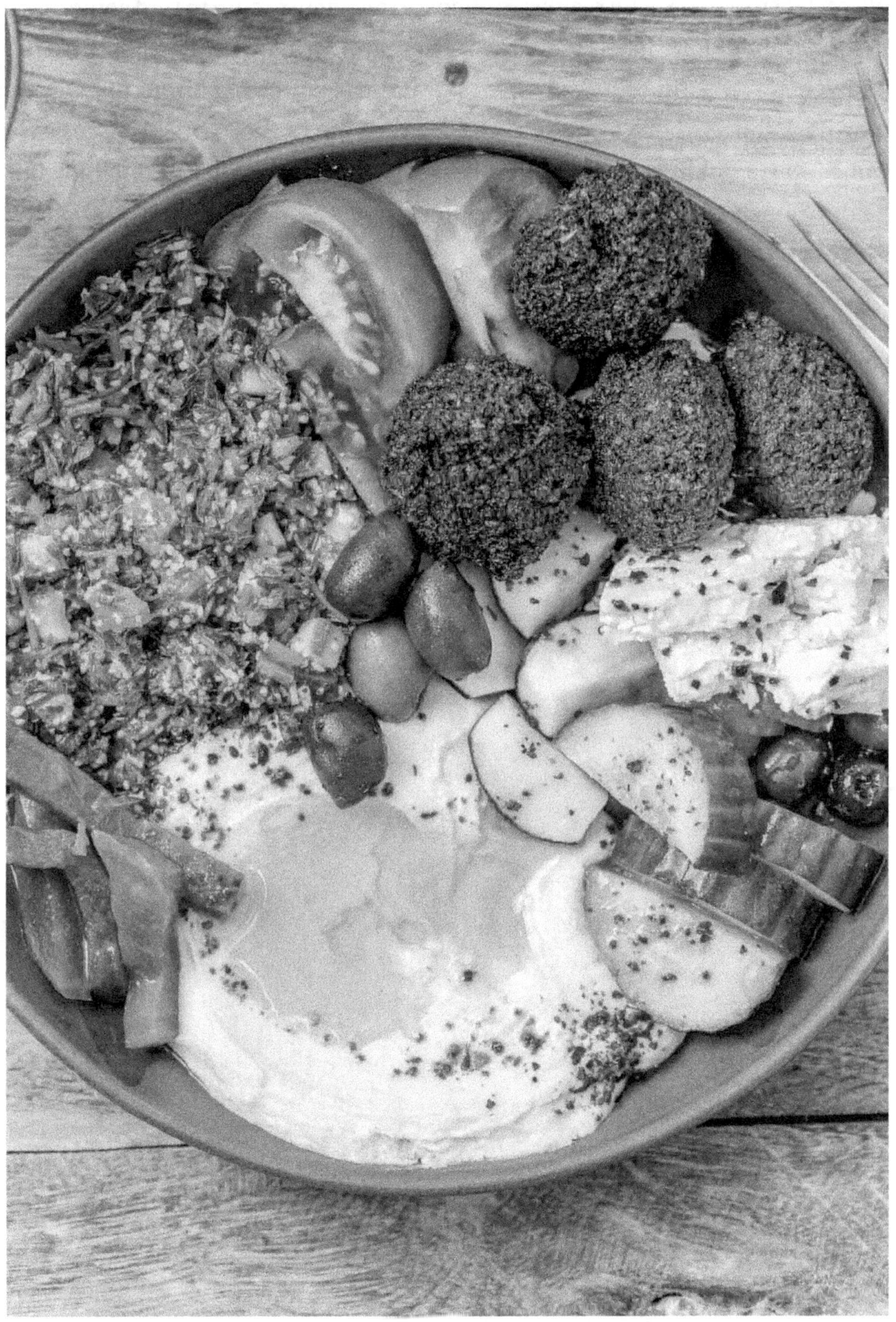

With 23 tasty and healthy recipes to choose from, you're sure to find something that fits your dietary needs and preferences. From grilled chicken Caesar salad and vegetarian chili to baked sweet potato fries and zucchini noodles with marinara sauce, there's something for everyone in this collection. So why wait? Start cooking up a storm and discover a new world of delicious and healthy meals that are sure to satisfy your cravings and nourish your body!

www.ingramcontent.com/pod-product-compliance
Lightning Source LLC
LaVergne TN
LVHW050347160826
845677LV00014B/3839